MAUREEN KENNEDY SALAMAN

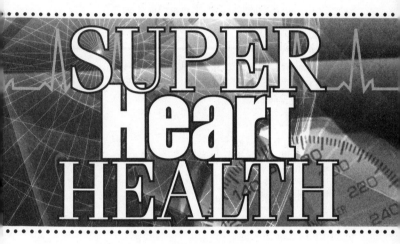

SUPER Heart HEALTH

Eliminating the Risk of

"The Quiet Killer," High Blood

Pressure, and Inflammation

STRATFORD
PUBLISHING

IMPORTANT NOTICE

This book is neither a medical guide nor a manual for self-treatment. It is instead intended as a reference work only. The information in this book is meant to help you make informed choices about your health, but is not intended as a substitute for any treatment that may be prescribed or recommended by your doctor or health care practitioner. If you should suspect that you suffer from a medical condition or problem, you should seek competent medical care without delay.

Super Heart Health: Eliminating the Risk of "The Quiet Killer,"
High Blood Pressure, and Inflammation
Copyright 2005
Maureen Kennedy Salaman

ISBN 0-913087-28-9
Second Printing

MKS, Inc.
1259 El Camino Real, Suite 1500
Menlo Park, California 94025
www.mksalaman.com
(650) 854-3922 telephone
(650) 854-5779 facsimile

Distributed by:
Maximum Living, Inc.
20071 Soulsbyville Road
Soulsbyville, California 95372-9748
www.maximizeyourlife.com
(209) 536-9300 telephone
(800) 445-4325 toll-free
(209) 536-9375 facsimile

All Scripture quotations, unless otherwise indicated, are taken from the *King James Version.*
Scripture quotations marked AMP are taken from *The Amplified Bible* (AMP). *The Amplified Bible, Old Testament.* Copyright © 1965, 1987 by The Zondervan Corporation. *The Amplified New Testament,* copyright © 1958, 1987 by The Lockman Foundation. Used by permission.

Literary development and interior and cover design by:
Koechel Peterson & Associates, Inc., Minneapolis, MN
Cover photo by Russ Fischella

Printed in the United States of America

CONTENTS

————— ∞ —————

To Margot and Harry DeWildt—
For how much your integrity,
judgment, and loyalty
have meant to me . . . and the world.
Your courage to stand for the truth
is a shining beacon in dark times.

Books by
Maureen Kennedy Salaman

⎯⎯⎯⎯⎯ ∞ ⎯⎯⎯⎯⎯

Foods That Heal

Foods That Heal Companion Cookbook

The Diet Bible

Nutrition: The Cancer Answer II

All Your Health Questions Answered Naturally II

How to Renew You:
The Complete Primer on Age Reversal

FOODS THAT HEAL

Achieving Super Immunity

The Renew You Diet

Super Heart Health

CHAPTER ONE

HIGH BLOOD PRESSURE— ELIMINATING THE RISK

*He who is stretched
like a rubber band will soon
find himself shooting
for the moon.*

—*Barbara Klein Moss*

BILL NEVER SAW THE KILLER sneak into his house and lie in wait. Next door Mary never once felt the killer's presence, though he lingered long. Down the same block Jack had no reason to think that a time bomb had invaded his life and was slowly ticking toward detonation.

Authorities warned them repeatedly that the killer was loose and that they were potential targets. But the killer is silent, invisible, and his name doesn't sound all that menacing. The consequences of disregard and ignorance can be lethal, though the killer can be stopped naturally.

The killer's name: High Blood Pressure. His alias: "The Silent Killer."

HYPERTENSION

There is a profound connection between high blood pressure—also called hypertension—and heart problems. Hypertension is called the "quiet killer" because often there are no obvious symptoms. The effect of long-term high blood pressure can include (1) weakening blood vessel walls; (2) aneurysms—abnormal expanding or hazardous ballooning of the artery wall that, when ruptured, can cause strokes, heart attacks, or instant death; and (3) congestive heart failure and kidney damage. A European study showed that having hypertension can increase the chances of dying of cardiovascular disease by 52 percent and of congestive heart failure by 63 percent.

Hypertension is defined as a blood pressure reading greater than 140 (systolic) over 90 (diastolic). Higher levels of either systolic or diastolic blood pressure are associated with an increased death rate, and these rates begin to rise at blood pressure levels as low as 120/80. An estimated 50 to 70 percent of elderly Americans have hypertension, and the risk of hypertension, at least in Americans, increases with age.

The first hint that hypertension is dietary-related arises when you examine the data from other countries. Not all populations experience this age-assumed increase in blood pressure. Population studies from nonagricultural societies suggest that average blood pressure does not, in fact, rise with age. In the United States, diastolic hypertension levels off at about age 55, but systolic hypertension continues to rise, even after age 80.

THE MINERAL ALLIANCE

People with consistent high blood pressure have

an increased stiffness, or resistance, in the peripheral arteries throughout the tissues of the body. This increased resistance causes the heart muscle to work harder, which can put a strain on the heart and circulatory system.

One of the most common conventional treatments for hypertension is calcium-channel blockers. They block calcium from attaching to the artery walls, causing them to stiffen. Adding magnesium to the diet will help overcome this issue, as magnesium helps relax muscles and dilate arteries, relieving high blood pressure. Magnesium also blocks calcium from entering soft tissues and causing them to become stiff.

One of the first things doctors recommend when confronted with someone who is hypertensive is to cut back on salt (sodium chloride). Be aware that salt comes from more than your saltshaker. If you read the labels on canned food items, you realize that most processed food has high levels of salt thanks to the age-old practice of using salt as a preservative.

The role of salt, or sodium, in high blood pressure is as controversial as it is widely accepted. Some say it has no effect; others say too much can severely increase blood pressure. However, if you look at the studies, you'll see a definite pattern. Tests that show no effect do not evaluate blood levels of the mineral potassium. Studies that consider potassium discover that too little potassium and too much salt cause dangerous hypertension.

A University of Pennsylvania study found that high blood pressure, as a result of a high salt diet, only occurred when patients had low blood levels of potassium.

One trial of 412 people with slightly elevated blood pressure found that a diet high in potassium, with just one-third the salt used in standard American fare, reduced their blood pressure by up to 11.5 points (millimeters of mercury) in 30 days. The diet was especially effective in African-Americans.

Sodium and potassium, in the correct ratio, regulate the body's fluid balance as well as increase heart strength. Heikki Karppanen, M.D., Department of Pharmacology and Toxicology, University of Helsinki, Finland, stated that it only takes a moderate restriction of sodium together with a high increase in potassium to lower blood pressure. Other research studies have shown that potassium alone, without considering the sodium issue, works to reduce blood pressure.

Just to clarify: eating too much salt does not cause high blood pressure. But if you don't get enough potassium in your diet and eat too much salt, you will increase your risk.

It's not enough to cut back on salt intake. First, you have to make sure you are getting enough minerals, especially potassium, in your food or through supplements. The minerals work together to ensure a healthy heart, with magnesium being the cornerstone of the equation. If you are low on magnesium and have too much calcium, it can result in the stiffening of the arteries. Not enough magnesium also results in inadequate amounts of potassium. Not enough potassium and salt takes effect, raising blood pressure.

It makes sense to include magnesium-rich foods in your diet. Better still, eliminate high-salt processed foods and choose God-given foods with the proper proportions of calcium, magnesium, and potassium, since they work together. These are wheat germ, sunflower seeds, soybeans, almonds, Brazil nuts, pistachios, and pecans. If you like trail mix, you're in luck. It's the best snack for a healthy heart.

Foods high in heart healthy magnesium are whole wheat, pumpkin seeds, millet, almonds, Brazil nuts, hazel nuts, dark-green vegetables, and molasses.

Potassium helps regulate blood pressure and may prevent strokes. A deficiency of this mineral is associated with irregular heartbeat and heart muscle damage. Foods high in potassium are blackstrap molasses, whole grains (a cup of millet has 980 mg), dried fruits (one cup of raisins has 1,362 mg), avocado (one = 1,204 mg), plantains (one cup = 739 mg), seeds (one cup of sunflower seeds = 1,334 mg) and nuts (one cup of pistachios = 1,399 mg).

A deficiency of another mineral, copper, has been associated with aneurysms. Copper is important for blood vessel strength and elasticity. Foods high in copper are seafood, nuts, beans, peas, molasses, and raisins.

If you are hypertensive, cut down on salt and eat these mineral-rich foods. Eliminate soft drinks. They contain high amounts of phosphorus, which rob your body of potassium. Watch how much sugar you eat as well, since it causes the body to retain sodium.

Remember, you're not what you put into your mouth; you're what you absorb and digest and deliver to cells. A tablet is only one to five percent absorbable. Since the process of digestion is a process of liquefaction, your body has to take a hard rock tablet and turn it into solution. This may not be possible due to a number of factors, such as inadequate stomach acid, food allergies, intestinal problems, and stress. When you are under stress, your stomach muscles tighten, further restricting digestion.

This is why it is so important that when you decide to supplement, you target minerals in solution—Maximum Living's MineralRich. It has the proper ratios of magnesium, calcium, and potassium, and includes vessel-strengthening copper.

STRESS-REDUCING NUTRIENTS

Stress happens. It's our body's response to fear or threat. But the body's reaction to it—high blood pressure, palpitations, and shock—can be reduced by adequate nutritional supplementation and faith.

Fear thou not; for I am with thee: be not dismayed; for I am thy God: I will strengthen thee; yea, I will help thee; yea, I will uphold thee with the right hand of my righteousness. —Isaiah 41:10; also see 1 Peter 4:12,13.

When problems, conflicts, and change threaten your peace of mind and blood pressure, turn to God first and receive His peace in your heart, then add nutritional supplementation. Stress causes the depletion of certain vitamins and minerals. High blood pressure, heart attacks, and strokes can be caused by constant stress. As stress creates deficiencies, a vicious cycle can occur.

Vitamin C—important in the inflammation equation—is the first vitamin to be used up during stress. All the B vitamins are next—used up in massive amounts. The body withdraws minerals to meet the demands of defense and breaks down protein from itself to create more hormones and antibodies. Your body's demand for calcium, magnesium, phosphorus, and potassium are also increased under stress.

Nutrients cushion the body's *response* to stress. You have to make life changes in order to reduce tension and pressure, but in the meantime, a daily supplement of Maximum Living's borage oil will help your body overcome its dangerous effects. Borage oil is high in linolenic acid, an essential fatty acid that inhibits abnormal adrenaline release and controls the body's impulse to raise blood pressure and increase the heart rate.

Researchers at the University of Waterloo, Ontario, Canada, found that when 30 men were randomly given three forms of essential fatty acids—fish oil, borage oil, and olive oil—only those receiving the borage oil did not have increased blood pressure or heart rate as a response to stress.

If I were asked to target any one stress-reducing vitamin, I would pinpoint all the B vitamins. There are no other nutrients more important to mental health than the B vitamins. The B-complex vitamins provide the body with energy, metabolizing fats and protein, and are necessary for the normal functioning of the nervous system.

If you could choose a food or supplement that would be the healthiest and most beneficial of all, it would be as close as possible to the way God made it. Every nutrient would be derived from natural sources, not synthesized. Next, it would include all the vitamins, minerals, and natural herbs that are needed for optimum health.

The most beneficial vitamin and mineral supplement on the market today is Maximum Living's Vita-Sprout. It contains all the nutrients discovered to be beneficial today, including freeze-dried sprouts, vegetables, and herbs. To make sure the entire complex of B vitamins are digested and assimilated properly, it includes friendly-body bacteria acidophilus. Nothing could be more complete for your immune system team than this power-packed, God-given formula.

HIGH BLOOD PRESSURE MISDIAGNOSED

Do you get anxious when you have to see a doctor? I know I do. The stress of going to a doctor can elevate your blood pressure. It is so common it has a name: white coat hypertension. One out of four people are estimated to have this syndrome, and as a result, many are misdiagnosed.

If you have been told you have high blood pressure, purchase a kit and take your blood pressure at home. This is important, too, when trying to determine what factors might be causing it: too much coffee/caffeine, smoking, anxiety, food allergies, or mineral deficiencies. If your blood pressure rises only when your mother-in-law visits, you don't need a prescription, you need a vacation.

If your blood pressure is taken using a cuff that is too small, you could have a higher blood pressure reading as a result. One classic study examined obese people already diagnosed with hypertension, then retook their blood pressure with the correct cuff for their arm circumference. Thirty-seven percent of them actually had normal blood pressure.

Recent research has shown that in large patients the subjects were 2.2 times more likely to be classified as hypertensive and 1.4 times more likely to be classified as borderline hypertensive when the standard cuff was used to measure blood pressure compared with the appropriately-sized large adult or thigh cuff. This was true even among people who were marginally large and whose arm circumferences were right around the cuff cutoff of about 13 inches. Using a cuff one size smaller than appropriate results in an incorrect diagnosis of hypertension approximately 36 percent of the time.

There are other factors besides cuff size that can

affect blood pressure readings. Improper technique when taking blood pressure has also been documented to affect blood pressure readings. This is especially true in pregnancy, where the threshold of intervention for borderline blood pressure is very low.

How many times have you had your blood pressure taken on the exam table with your legs dangling and back unsupported? This is incorrect and shockingly common. According to Charlene Grim, RN (chairwoman of the American Heart Association Committee that reviewed the current blood pressure guidelines), taking a person's blood pressure when seated on the exam table with no back support can raise blood pressure by 10 points.

Another common technique, pumping the cuff too high at the beginning of the blood pressure measurement, also raises blood pressure. This can result in what is termed "cuff inflation hypertension." This can be a problem for plus-sized women, because medical personnel often assume that all heavy people have high blood pressure and accordingly pump the cuff up quite high at the start.

To take a person's blood pressure accurately, the patient should be: seated with legs supported, back supported, legs uncrossed, and without the arms resting on the armrests of the chair (the nurse should support the arm for you to the correct height).

COMING ATTRACTIONS

You should feel better about Silent Killer now that you know there is much you can do to stop him from endangering your health. Read the following chapters and enjoy enlightenment as it brings you out of the dark ages of fear so you can feel confident that you will enjoy Super Heart Health the rest of your life.

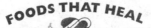

CHAPTER TWO

A SEISMIC SHIFT IN HEART CARE

> *I know of no more encouraging fact than the unquestionable ability of man to elevate his life by conscious endeavor. To affect the quality of the day, that is the highest of arts.*
>
> —Henry David Thoreau

WHEN IT COMES TO UNDERSTANDING heart health, most of us feel as overwhelmed as Dorothy when she approached the mighty Wizard of Oz. Medical expressions and nomenclature, such as arteriosclerosis, cardiovascular disease, heart attacks, heart failure, arrhythmia, coronary artery disease, hypertension, hypercholesteremia, hyperlipidemia, valvular stenosis, and tachycardia, thunder and intimidate and make us feel helpless. We need to pull the veil back and expose the Wizard and his fancy words. They only describe basic, commonsense concepts of blood flow, artery strength, blood quality, and heart muscle strength.

Rest assured: you can understand. Let me simplify it by outlining the seismic shift that has occurred in heart care.

CHOLESTEROL IS NOT THE MAIN PROBLEM

In the '70s, the *Wall Street Journal* introduced the cholesterol frenzy with the headline, "The Age of Cholesterol Dawns for Food Manufacturers and Pharmaceuticals." The article went on to say that cholesterol is not a main factor for heart attacks, which was a bold declaration at a time when massive corporate marketing campaigns were proclaiming the opposite.

Because high cholesterol is often found at the scene of heart problems, it gets blamed for the problems. That's as logical as blaming ambulances for car accidents because they are often found at the scene of the accidents. The fact is that many people with high cholesterol live perfectly healthy lives, with no heart disease. Some very sick people, with AIDs, cancer, and heart disease, can have very low cholesterol.

Much empirical evidence proves that artificially lowering cholesterol is dangerous because we need cholesterol to manufacture sex hormones, vitamin D, DHEA, and cell membranes. Cholesterol is needed to protect the body against stress. Lowering cholesterol artificially affects mental acuity and severely disables the ability to cope with physical and mental stress. Studies have shown a three- to 13-fold rise in violent deaths among people taking cholesterol-lowering drugs.

THE LOST PUZZLE PIECE—INFLAMMATION

What have I learned that you need to know? *Inflammation is the top risk factor for heart attacks, not cholesterol.* Having read the brilliant work of Dr. Valentin Fuster, President of the American Heart Association and director of the Cardiovascular Institute at Mount Sinai School of Medicine in New York, I was the lone voice getting the word out. In his book, *The Vulnerable Atherosclerotic Plaque*, he states that inflammation—not high cholesterol—is the issue of importance.

Now the establishment press has jumped on the bandwagon. As of this writing, the most recent report on this issue was a *Time* magazine (January 23, 2005) cover story heralding inflammation as the hidden cause of heart disease, cancer, and Alzheimer's.

Hardly a week goes by without the publication of yet another study uncovering a new way that chronic inflammation does harm to the body. It destabilizes cholesterol deposits in the coronary arteries, leading to heart attacks and strokes. It chews up nerve cells in the brains of Alzheimer's victims. It even encourages the mutation of cells into cancer. In other words, chronic inflammation may be the engine that drives many of the most feared illnesses of middle and old age.

Inflammation in circulating blood triggers heart attacks and strokes by activating blood-clotting mechanisms, which in turn can slow down or stop blood flow. Inflammation is the body's natural response to injury, and blood clotting is part of that response. It is estimated that between 25 million and 35 million healthy middle-aged Americans have normal cholesterol but above-average inflammation.

Old and new research shows that childhood diseases, as well as poor lifestyle choices, create this inflammatory risk. Eliminating childhood diseases may be a huge step in preventing adult heart disease. In one fascinating historical study, U.S. Civil War veterans who had an infectious disease as young men were more likely to have heart disease after age 50. Even frequent diarrhea during infancy, a sign of infection, is linked to cardiovascular disease in adulthood. Experts estimate that Americans now in their 50s are 15 percent more likely to have cardiovascular disease if they had a serious infectious disease in childhood.

Low birth weight is indicted in the case against inflammation. A study found that men who weighed less than 5.5 pounds at birth have, on average, a 50 percent greater chance of dying of heart disease than men with a higher birth weight. Women born weighing less than 5.5 pounds have a 23 percent greater risk of cardiovascular disease than women born larger. The reason: a lack of proper nutrition in the cells and organs of the low birth weight baby. A lack of vitamin B12 and folic acid in the preemie can adversely affect how the liver effectively filters blood and regulates blood pressure. Cells wear out faster, causing a rise in blood pressure and the heart disease that typically follows.

Poor lifestyle choices, such as smoking, poor diet, and a lack of exercise, create a lifetime of irritation, injury, healing, and reinjury to the inside of the blood vessels, which can cause small arterial plaque deposits to suddenly rupture like popcorn kernels, choking off the blood supply to the heart. The plaque itself can become inflamed as white blood cells invade in a misguided autoimmune defense attempt.

Inflammation from all sources—prenatal, postnatal, and lifetime—produces molecular evidence that can be identified through laboratory testing. One such "inflammatory molecule" is C-reactive protein. Brigham and Women's Hospital studies showed that measuring C-reactive protein levels can help predict the risk of heart attack in postmenopausal women and middle-aged men.

YOU DON'T NEED A MAGIC PILL

The race is on to uncover the key molecular triggers of artery inflammation and develop ways to detect and treat it before it does fatal damage. Virtually every pharmaceutical company is working on a "magic pill" to limit inflammation.

However, we don't need a magic pill because we have the benefit of knowledge—information on natural anti-inflammatories and supplements that reduce the damage the body's immune system exacts when battling infection. Fortunately for us, there are many nutrients capable of raising "good guy" HDL cholesterol, reducing inflammation, strengthening the heart muscles, and lowering high blood pressure. Read along while I show you which, and how they work.

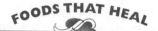

CHAPTER THREE

NUTRIENTS FOR INFLAMMATION RECOVERY

*Feed me
with the food
that is needful
for me.*

—*Proverbs 30:8 AMP*

WHAT IS A MOSQUITO'S favorite sport? Skin diving.

As anyone suffering itching mosquito bites can attest, inflammation can be irritating at best.

But is it always bad? Inflammation is the body's immune system response to the presence of a foreign substance or injury. It stops bleeding, heals injured tissue, and kills bacteria. Inflammation is the most potent effect of the immune defense when the body is injured. However, as we move away from natural foods, live in synthetic environments, and breathe toxic air, our immune systems are overloaded, and chronic inflammation results. Nature has provided a good protective strategy in the inflammatory process, but it is forced to go too far too often.

Many of the serious, chronic, and unsolved diseases

that plague our modern civilization are inflammatory disorders. As a result, much of conventional medical therapy is directed at controlling inflammation. Now we can add heart disease to the list. Studies in the past few years have shown that inflammation plays a role in atherosclerosis, the buildup of fatty deposits in blood vessels that can lead to heart attacks, strokes, and other cardiovascular problems.

Now that well-informed experts agree that inflammation is a bigger threat to your heart than cholesterol, what can you do about it? Follow along while I give you the latest research on how to use diet and supplementation to reduce inflammation.

FOODS THAT FIGHT INFLAMMATION

Eating certain foods help fight inflammation because they contain power-packed nutrients. If you target foods and take supplements that contain these active ingredients, you create a one-two punch for super heart health.

Eat fish. It's the fatty oil in fish that makes it so heart healthy. Fish oil is an omega-3 fatty acid. In areas where fish consumption is high, such as Japan, Greenland, and the areas bordering the Mediterranean Sea, people eat considerably more fish than in the U.S. They also have a much lower risk for cardiovascular disease. Fish with the highest amounts of omega-3 are: Atlantic mackerel, albacore tuna, Atlantic herring, chinook salmon, lake trout, Atlantic salmon, and bluefin tuna. It is recommended that we eat fish two to three times a week.

Eat berries. Colorful foods, such as berries, have the highest amounts of bioflavonoids, substances proven to reduce inflammation. Berries contain the most, but bioflavonoids are also present in colorful fruits and vegetables. An article in the medical journal *The Lancet* found that bioflavonoids effectively reduce the histamine reaction common in allergy reactions.

Eat onions. One bioflavonoid in particular, quercetin, is so powerful it is compared to Cromolyn, a prescription antihistamine. Quercetin is found in yellow and red onions.

I don't advocate alcohol, but recent studies show that people who *drink red wine in moderation* (a glass a day) have less heart problems. Grapes and fermented grapes, especially those used for red wine, contain vast amounts of anti-inflammatory bioflavonoids. In a study at the Medical University of South Carolina in Charleston, non-drinkers showed one-third more inflammation than low to moderate drinkers. Get the flavonoids without the alcohol by eating red grapes or drinking grape juice.

Learn to appreciate spicy food. Cayenne pepper, tumeric, garlic, and ginger are all noted inflammation reducers. Garlic only works when raw (or supplemented). Try chopped raw garlic in Chinese ginger salad or try pickled garlic. Tumeric has been used in both the Indian and Chinese systems of medicine (and their food) for the treatment of many forms of inflammation. Its anti-inflammatory properties are likened to the pharmaceutical effects of hydrocortisone and phenylbutazone, only much safer. It is the bioflavonoids in curcumin, which gives tumeric its yellow color, that has been found in studies to work better than even Ibuprofen, a popular over-the-counter pain medicine.

Become a vegetarian. Not only are fruits, grains, and vegetables better for you, too much high-protein meat can increase inflammation. Researchers at the Fleming Heart and Health Institute in Omaha found that when people ate a high-protein diet for a year, blood vessel inflammation jumped 62 percent and coronary artery disease worsened. If you can't do without meat, choose animals that have been range fed. Grass contains omega-3 fatty acids, while corn does not.

Don't cook meat on high heat. If you broil, make it fish. Grilling, broiling, and frying meat and poultry create damaged proteins called AGEs (advanced glycosylation end products) that trigger inflammation. In diabetics who ate a high AGE-inducing diet, inflammation jumped 35 percent. Mount Sinai School of Medicine researchers discovered it dropped 20 percent in those on low AGE-inducing diets. To reduce AGEs, poach or boil chicken, and eat more fish. Broiled fish has about one-fourth the AGEs of broiled steak or chicken. Fruits and vegetables are low in AGEs; cheeses are high in them.

NUTRIENTS THAT FIGHT INFLAMMATION

Isolating the "active ingredients" in food that encourage health and overcome heart disease is what turned the health food movement into the alternative health movement. Now, instead of turning to pharmaceuticals, the educated look to supplements that do the same thing naturally and safely.

NSAIDs, or Non-Steroidal Anti-Inflammatory Drugs, are prescription and over-the-counter painkillers recommended by doctors and promoted extensively for all kinds of inflammation, from arthritis to bruises. Some are considered anti-inflammatory; some only kill the pain. Unfortunately, NSAIDs do a lot more—they increase the risk of bleeding ulcers and corrode the stomach lining. To counter this side effect, researchers are now targeting nutrients that protect against the effect of NSAIDs. Doctors in Spain found that supplementing with the mineral zinc increased protective mucous and strengthened cells.

THE MINERAL SOLUTION

Zinc also helps reduce inflammation. During stress or inflammation there is a reduction in zinc concentrations in certain tissues and a redistribution of zinc internally. An article in the *Journal of the American College of Nutrition* stated that head injury patients who received zinc supplementation had better healing compared to those who received a placebo.

Another mineral with anti-inflammatory properties is selenium. In studies, selenium has been shown to be particularly effective for rheumatoid arthritis, as it increases oxygenation in synovial tissues in joint spaces, where inflammation occurs.

I will discuss more about minerals in the next chapter, in relation to your heart muscles. For a holistic approach to heart health, I use Maximum Living's MineralRich, which is a daily supplement that provides all the minerals in the proper proportions, including trace minerals, your body needs, along with vitamins B12 and biotin . . . all in a delicious liquid that will be rapidly absorbed by your body. Thousands of people use this remarkable product daily to ensure their immune system is in peak fighting condition.

VEGETARIANS EAT MORE ENZYMES

In one study, death from heart disease was 57 percent lower in vegetarians than the general population. Vegetarians eat more fiber, less fat, and are generally more conscientious about their health. However, one factor is very important to consider. Vegetarians eat more enzymes because fruits, vegetables, and grains—particularly when raw—have the most. Enzymes are the compounds you need to break down food into nutrients. When you eat right, they are plentiful and digestion is thorough. When they are lacking, so is your health.

Bromelain, the enzyme found in pineapple, is recommended when joints, muscles, or ligaments are swollen and inflamed. Since you would have to eat two whole pineapples a day to achieve this anti-inflammatory effect, it's good we have supplemental formulas with bromelain.

If you are a meat lover, this bit of information should make you happy. While too much protein encourages inflammation, this can be overcome to a certain extent by supplemental proteolytic enzymes, which specifically digest protein. One such enzyme is papain, which is isolated from papaya.

When we get enough enzymes to digest food and have enough left over to patrol the body, they enter the bloodstream—are called "free floating"—and become potent anti-inflammatories. When they are missing, the body's natural inflammatory immune response can become chronic. Enzymes have been used clinically to treat the inflammation and edema that typically follow oral surgery.

If you are eating a lot of protein, or have a family history of heart disease, circulation problems, or strokes, take digestive enzymes with your meals in a supplement formula such as Maximum Living's Multi-Enzyme. Include Maximum Living's free-floating enzyme formula Enzyme Ease, which is coated, so the enzymes move through your stomach and are released into the bloodstream—free-floating—where they can prevent chronic inflammation.

If you are interested in learning more about this, read my award-winning book *Nutrition: The Cancer Answer II*. It was voted the best health book in the U.S. and has won awards in Great Britain, Australia, and the Philippines. There is a whole chapter on enzymes, and it is still the best information out there.

AN OILY SOLUTION

I already explained why eating fish is so important, and the fact that fish contains omega-3 fatty acids. For supplemental omega-3 fatty acid, I take Maximum Living's flaxseed oil gel capsules. Flaxseed oil contains 50 to 60 percent omega-3 fatty acids—almost twice as much as fish oil. Another term you might have heard is PUFAs—polyunsaturated fatty acids. They are the healthy kinds of fats—as opposed to saturated fats. Essential fatty acids are PUFAs.

Another kind of supplemental essential fatty acid is omega-6, found in seeds and seed oils. The best source is gamma-linolenic acid (GLA) from borage oil. GLA is an excellent anti-inflammatory. In one study, when nine borage seed oil capsules were given daily to arthritic volunteers for 12 weeks, there was a substantial reduction in prostaglandins and leukotrienes, alleviating their painful arthritic symptoms. Finally, borage oil is more bioavailable. In other words, the body more readily accepts it. Take Maximum Living borage oil, while reducing NSAID dosage, and continue afterward.

SUPPLEMENTAL ANTI-INFLAMMATORY FORMULA

If you have arthritis or know someone who has, you've probably heard of glucosamine sulfate. Because arthritis is caused by inflammation, this information is of value. Maximum Living offers an arthritis formula called Joint Assure that contains many potent anti-inflammatory ingredients. It includes the enzymes bromelain and curcumin, as well as cayenne pepper. Also included is feverfew, a medicinal herb used to prevent the inflammation that precedes migraines; and yucca root, which is known to reduce inflammation and obstructions of the joints.

Continue to follow along to the next chapter as I discuss the nutrients important to your heart's muscle mass—the cardiac muscle.

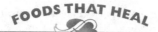

CHAPTER FOUR

MINERALS FOR MUSCLE STRENGTH

> *I wish above all things that thou*
> *mayest prosper and be in health,*
> *even as thy soul prospereth.*
>
> —3 John 1:2

LOUIS PASTEUR ONCE SAID, "The more I study nature, the more I am amazed at the Creator." I have been struck by the same reality whenever I consider the human heart in all its intricacies and complexities.

Make a fist. That's how big your heart is. It's not very big, is it? What do we know about the heart—the actual heart organ?

The heart is essentially a mass of pumping muscle. It is efficient, and it is designed to never stop pumping. From the moment of its development in the fetal body through the moment of death, the heart contracts and relaxes, pushing blood through its chambers and into your arteries, veins, and capillaries.

The heart beats an average 70 times per minute, 100,000 times a day, 36.5 million times a year, and 2.5 billion times in a 68-year lifetime. Approximately 2.5 ounces of blood are pumped through the heart with every heartbeat. Every day it pumps 1,080 gallons of blood.

The heart is central to your circulatory system. It is your workhorse, your internal brawn, the strength of your body system. When you run, your heart pumps more quickly. When you sleep, your heart pumps more slowly. It must be strong or you will be weak.

WHEN YOUR HEART IS NOT STRONG

Doctors use the term *cardiomyopathy* to describe what happens when your heart muscle is not strong enough to function properly. They call the muscle of your heart the myocardium (even though the heart *is* a muscle).

Cardiomyopathy—heart weakness—is blamed on inflammation. The three types of cardiomyopathy—dilated, hypertrophic, and restrictive—are defined based on how the heart is affected by inflammation. In the first, the heart muscle becomes weak and the heart chambers dilate. In the second, the heart muscle is much thicker than normal. In the third, the heart becomes stiff, and its chambers cannot adequately fill with blood.

Cardiomyopathy causes congestive heart failure, abnormal heart rhythms (arrhythmias and murmurs), blood clots (slower-moving blood encourages clotting), high blood pressure readings, narrowed arteries, obstructed blood flow, mitral (heart) valve leakage, and angina (chest pain or discomfort caused by reduced blood supply to the heart muscle).

The reasons for why inflammation occurs is important. In some cases, nutritional deficiencies can be blamed. In other cases, viruses and illnesses are the cause. Nutritional supplementation can help with both. Knowing how to nourish your heart muscle and knowing what is necessary for a healthy heart are essential.

It was long assumed that when the heart is damaged—such as after a heart attack—the damage is permanent. This assumption has been challenged by researchers with the National Heart, Lung, and Blood Institute, a component of the National Institutes of Health, and the National Institute on Aging. Now we know that healing can take place in a damaged heart. A weak heart can become a healthy heart.

MAGNESIUM FOR A MAGNIFICENT MUSCLE

I have never seen such a rush to evaluate any nutrient for heart problems as regards magnesium over the past few decades. First, doctors and researchers saw the evidence. It was so compelling they couldn't ignore it. Then they tentatively, cautiously, and reluctantly conducted more trials. Finally, a large-scale study was conducted over several years to demonstrate, once and for all, its efficacy. Magnesium has survived these trials and has made it through the gate with flying colors.

For the past 50 years, doctors have successfully used magnesium in the treatment of cardiac arrhythmias, which can occur when the heart muscle isn't strong enough to pump blood. At the Royal Hobart Hospital in Southern Australia, researchers added one single nutrient, magnesium, to the nutritional intake of patients with any kind of heart problem, including angina, arrhythmia, and heart attack. That year the death rate among heart patients admitted to the hospital went from 30 percent to one percent.

Two randomized trials showed patients treated with intravenous magnesium following a heart attack were less likely to die, and that it reduced the frequency of arrhythmias. Editors of the medical journal *The Lancet* stated that "the reduction in arrhythmias and deaths in magnesium-treated patients is a real and substantial finding."

Dr. Mildred S. Seelig, American College of Nutrition, believes that a deficiency of magnesium can cause heart problems. She maintains that when people with cardiovascular problems and low magnesium intake try to improve their health with strenuous exercise, such as jogging, they could be endangering their health. Magnesium requirements are markedly increased during physical stress, and the heart is much more susceptible to arrhythmias during physical exertion if the body's magnesium level is low.

During my television show, *Making Healthy Choices*, Michael Schachter, M.D., agreed, stating that many cases of sudden heart attacks during stressful exercise can be directly attributed to a magnesium deficiency.

Important to remember is that magnesium must be balanced with calcium and potassium for the proper regulation of heart muscle contraction. Researchers at a heart institute in Israel found that potassium levels were severely low among patients with heart arrhythmias, as compared to those who did not have arrhythmias, concluding in the *International Journal of Cardiology* that potassium is an important factor in the development of arrhythmias.

THE CALCIUM/MAGNESIUM CONNECTION

The most fascinating thing about magnesium is the fact that it moves calcium out of the tissues and into the bones, where it is needed, or into urine, where it is excreted if the body has too much. It is this calcium-blocking effect that makes magnesium so protective of the heart.

Dr. R. M. Touyz, of South Africa, believes the addition of magnesium in a treatment program for high blood pressure would decrease the need for calcium channel blockers and their subsequent side effects.

If we are lacking calcium, magnesium will be depleted. Not enough magnesium results in calcium being deposited in soft tissue and arteries. One type of cardiomyopathy is the stiffening of the heart muscle. This may occur, since inadequate magnesium causes calcium to be deposited in the heart muscle.

It's not just magnesium and calcium. For optimum health, we need all the minerals in balance. Like the slats of a barrel, they work together to keep the heart whole, flexible, and strong. The ratio of all the minerals together is just as important.

The typical American diet, low in greens and high in dairy products, brings the calcium/magnesium ratio to five calcium to every one magnesium, above the four to one ratio of Finland, which has the highest incidence of heart disease in young to middle-aged men.

Finnish researchers, desperate for answers to their epidemic of heart problems, hit on the magnesium/calcium answer. Veterinarian and medical doctor Dr. H. Korpela, at the Department of Human Health, University of Kuopio, Finland, examined 18 pigs that had died of sudden heart failure. He found low concentrations of magnesium and high levels of calcium in their heart muscles and livers, as compared to healthy pigs and those that died of other diseases.

Once again, we're back to Maximum Living's MineralRich. The research scientists who formulated MineralRich looked at the heart and the other body systems and used the ratios most opportunistic for the body. The calcium/magnesium ratio in MineralRich is exactly what is needed for strong heart muscles and smooth-flowing blood. It also contains zinc, copper, and selenium, three antioxidant minerals that according to research help prevent heart problems from occurring in the first place.

AMINO ACIDS FOR MUSCLE STRENGTH

From the pages of sports medicine come the most widely-used supplements to boost muscle strength: amino acids. When amino acids are lost or missing, muscle tissue breaks down. While vitamin E can reverse this process—as I'll discuss in the next chapter—amino acids can prevent it from happening in the first place.

The story starts with protein. Your heart muscle is made up of protein. Protein is composed of approximately 22 amino acids. All but eight can be produced in the human body; the rest have to be obtained from food or supplements. If just one amino acid is low or missing, even temporarily, protein synthesis will fall or stop altogether, and the heart muscle can become weak.

Athletes incorporate amino acid formulas in their daily nutritional routine, especially after injury, to rebuild muscle. Amino acids help prevent the body from breaking down protein in injured muscles, such as a heart damaged by inflammation.

For full supplemental benefit, look for an amino acid formula that includes all the free-form amino acids, such as Maximum Living's amino acid formula, which is all natural and derived from a hypoallergenic whey source to avoid food allergy complications. The following heart muscle amino acids are included in this formula:

- L-Proline is a major component of heart muscle and is lost when the heart is injured or under stress.
- L-Arginine is a precursor to nitric oxide, which signals the smooth muscles in the blood vessels to relax and dilate, allowing blood to flow more freely and lowering blood pressure. It eases the symptoms and pains of angina as well. Researchers at Einstein Medical School in New York City found that, after moderate surgery, people who received an extra 15 grams of arginine a day had a 60 percent reduction in protein loss compared to patients who did not receive the supplement.

SOY PROTEIN APPROVED BY FDA

Protein is important to healthy heart muscle, but protein needs proteolytic enzymes to be digested. Meat does not contain proteolytic enzymes, robbing us of the free-flowing enzymes that guard us against cancer, heart disease, Alzheimer's, and inflammation, which causes heart problems. Proteolytic enzymes are abundant in vegetable proteins such as soy.

Soy has been found so beneficial that the Food and Drug Administration (FDA) has given food manufacturers permission to claim that soy protein food products help lower the risk of heart disease. This does not apply to soy supplements, only foods that contain soy protein.

There is a natural, nutritionally complete soy protein snack product I am very excited about. It's called Maximum Living Nutrition Bites, and I love the taste and smooth, chewy consistency. They have all the nutrients necessary to build lean muscle, help burn cholesterol, and restore the body to optimum health. It is packaged as chewy nuggets and comes in three flavors: chocolate, vanilla nut, and peanut butter, with more delicious flavors coming.

Maximum Living Nutrition Bites have all of the good stuff and none of the bad stuff. The soy protein in these tasty snacks contains many vital nutrients, including fat-reducing enzymes, essential fatty acids, nitrogen, and amino acids. And this soy is non-GMO, meaning it is certified as non-genetically modified or manipulated. Unlike most products like it, they contain no hydrogenated oils or refined sugar.

Captain Dennis Donegan of the Special Forces in Afghanistan and Iraq reported that he found the muscle-sustaining strength to endure intense firefights, battles, and extreme exertion with Maximum Living Nutrition Bites.

WHEN THE DAMAGE IS DONE

In this booklet you've discovered that many heart problems are associated with inflammation, and what you can do to limit it. You've learned how to increase the strength of your heart muscle, and how to avoid chronic, consistent high blood pressure so it doesn't cause permanent damage to vital organs.

However, there are so many factors that affect heart health—stress, chemicals, air pollution, genetics, deficiencies, poor lifestyle choices, and illnesses—that damage control is also important. The next chapter will explain what you can do to protect your heart when living takes a backseat to surviving.

CHAPTER FIVE
DAMAGE CONTROL

> *The amount of antioxidants*
> *you maintain in your body*
> *is directly proportional*
> *to how long you will live.*
>
> —*Richard Cutler, M.D.,*
> *National Institutes of Health*

OBVIOUSLY, WHOEVER CLAIMED, "The best things in life are free," didn't know about *free radicals*. They're free all right, but they're one of the worst things in life. Just in case the only free radicals you have ever heard of were Abby Hoffman and Jerry Rubin back in the '60s, let's take a look at them by way of studying antioxidants.

"Antioxidants" are nutrients in foods and herbs that retard oxidation, helping prevent the deterioration of cell membranes that naturally occur over time. Because they characteristically prevent cell breakdown, they also keep delicate arterial membranes flexible and strong, and heart muscle intact. They are also part of the body's defense system, helping to minimize damage when injury occurs.

Antioxidants are viable, valuable, and an effective means of not only preventing heart disease but also reducing tissue damage and encouraging healing when heart problems occur. In 2004, 30 percent of Americans were taking some form of antioxidant supplement, according to the American Heart Association.

ANTIOXIDANTS BANISH FREE RADICALS

Antioxidants are our way of warding off the damaging effects of time by stopping the formation of free radicals—wayward molecules that steal electrons in order to form pairs. This electron-stripping is referred to as oxidation. Oxidation is what rusts metal, makes oils rancid, and turns a sliced apple brown—so imagine what it does to your body! Free radicals also cause the heart muscle to deteriorate over time, making it more susceptible to damage in the event of arrhythmias and blockages.

While our individual cells are capable of fighting destructive free radicals, they need help from antioxidants. In a Canadian survey of over 2,200 men, it was found that those who had been taking antioxidant vitamins reduced the risk of death from heart disease by 78 percent, cutting their risk of a heart attack by 58 percent and reducing their risk of angina (spasm of the coronary artery) by 15 percent.

Large amounts of antioxidants are required. Vitamins A, C, E, beta carotene, selenium, zinc, copper, coenzyme Q10, and garlic extract are the important ones. Each has a special cell-protective or regenerating function. For example, vitamins A, C, and E team up to protect blood vessels and other body tissues from free radical damage.

In one study, researchers exposed red blood cells to destructive ultraviolet light, some with vitamin E added. Those without vitamin E aged faster than those with this essential antioxidant. Further, the unprotected red blood cells bulged like an over-inflated bicycle tire, while those with vitamin E resisted the reaction far longer, demonstrating that vitamin E's antioxidant action extends cell life and, therefore, human life.

Recent studies show that vitamin E helps prevent heart disease. Researchers at the University of Southern California School of Medicine found that heart patients who took 100 IU of vitamin E plus niacin had fewer heart problems over two years than those who did not take the vitamins. In "The Physicians Health Study," more than 20,000 doctors discovered that vitamin E protected their patients against heart disease.

The British medical journal *The Lancet* published the results of a study of 2,000 patients with coronary heart disease. Half the patients received 400 to 800 IU of vitamin E daily and were found to have a 75 percent reduction in heart attacks.

Antioxidants work in virtually all aspects of heart disease. They help blood circulation, inhibit blood platelets from sticking together, and reduce plaque in the arteries. Most study findings support the hypothesis that antioxidant vitamins may reduce the risk of coronary artery disease and subsequent heart problems.

"The Nurses Health Study," which began in 1976 with a group of 90,000 participants without heart disease, showed that 16 years later those with the highest risk of heart disease were those with the lowest intake of beta carotene and vitamins E and C. In the highest beta carotene group, there was a 22 percent reduction in the risk of heart problems, compared to the lowest group. There was a 34 percent reduction in risk of heart problems among women taking the most vitamin E. All in all, people taking the most antioxidants had a 50 percent reduction in the likelihood of ending up in the hospital with a heart attack.

In "The Scottish Heart Health Study," over 10,000 middle-aged men were evaluated for their intake of vitamins C and E and beta carotene. It was found that these antioxidants had a highly protective effect on their hearts. Critically evaluating the study data was Susan Todd of the Department of Applied Statistics. She concluded in the *Journal of Clinical Epidemiology* that the study was valid, and that, indeed, it appears that antioxidant vitamin intake protects against coronary heart disease in men.

One kind of heart problem has been directly linked to a deficiency of the mineral selenium, a particularly potent antioxidant. Keshan's disease was first discovered in Keshan County in the Heilongjiang Province of China, where it was rampant in 1935. Once it was discovered that selenium deficiency was the underlying cause of the disease and selenium supplementation could prevent it, it stopped being a major public health problem.

Ever wonder why so many people have heart attacks in hospitals? Here's one possible explanation. An article in *Clinical Chemistry* states that patients who are fed intravenously in the hospital may have dangerously low levels of selenium, enough to increase their risk of a heart attack.

Copper and zinc are two minerals noted for their antioxidant and healing properties. They work together, and a deficiency of one will create a deficiency in the other. Denis M. Medeiros, Ph.D., R.D., of the Department of Human Nutrition, College of Human Ecology, Ohio State University, Columbus, found animals fed low-copper diets may develop cardiac abnormalities. High blood cholesterol is also associated with copper deficient diets. In rat experiments, copper deficient diets have resulted in heart problems.

Studies at the Cincinnati Medical Center and Institute of Environmental Health in Ohio have concluded that the body's intake and ability to absorb zinc and copper appear to be significant factors in preventing both cardiomyopathy, a degenerative disease of the heart muscle that can cause heart failure, and angiopathy, a degeneration of small arteries that can impede blood flow. An article in *Science News* reports that the diets of many in the United States are deficient in one or both of these essential trace minerals.

Researchers at Loma Linda University School of Medicine, Department of Microbiology, studied garlic and found that its major component, S-allyl cysteine, is a potent free radical scavenger, helping to protect heart cells from oxidative injury.

Another antioxidant proven to help the heart is coenzyme Q10, a powerful antioxidant that helps fight congestive heart failure (CHF), a common condition in which the heart becomes too weak to pump enough blood to the tissues of the body. Because of this pumping action failure, blood returning to the heart backs up, leading to a buildup of fluid in the lungs. This "waterlogging" of the lungs causes weakness and shortness of breath.

In a study from Japan, 17 patients with mild congestive heart failure (CHF) were given 30 mg/day of coenzyme Q10. Every patient improved within four weeks, and 53 percent became completely symptom-free. Coenzyme Q10 has also been found to help people with severe CHF. In a double-blind study, 641 such patients were given either coenzyme Q10 or a placebo for one year. The number of patients requiring hospitalization for worsening heart failure was 38 percent less in the coenzyme Q10 group than in the control group. In another study, the survival rate nearly tripled when patients with severe CHF were given the nutrient.

AN APPLE A DAY KEEPS THE DOCTOR AWAY

In nature, foods highest in vitamin C also contain large amounts of bioflavonoids, which aid their anti-oxidant properties and work against inflammation. In a five-year study of 805 Dutch men between the ages of 65 and 84, it was found that those who consumed the most foods containing bioflavonoids—apples, other fruit, berries, garlic, onions, and green tea leaves—suffered half as many fatal heart attacks as men who consumed the lowest amounts. Men who had a higher intake of bioflavonoids had a lower risk of death from coronary heart disease and of having a first heart attack, reported Dr. Michael Hertog in an article in *The Lancet*. Hertog credited eating one large apple a day with a high intake of flavonoids.

Garlic itself has proven to have many heart-smart properties, no doubt in part due to its bioflavonoids. People who enjoy the zestful cuisine of southern Europe have fewer fatal heart attacks than do those in the north, where the food is blander. Among the benefits of the hearty Mediterranean diet is the consumption of large amounts of garlic. Now, this culinary tradition is being hailed by scientists as one of the reasons Americans should look to their European cousins for mealtime tips.

In eight different studies, people given daily garlic or garlic extract lowered their cholesterol levels by an average of nine percent. Some investigators have also found a rise in protective HDL-cholesterol. In addition, something in garlic keeps platelets from being sticky, so they are less able to clump together to form a clot when a blood vessel is injured. And garlic has been discovered to step up the ordinarily low level of clot-dissolving (fibrinolytic) activity present in blood, an action that favors the breakdown of any clot that did develop.

SUPPLEMENTING YOUR ANTIOXIDANT ARSENAL

Life is like a box of chocolates. You never really know what you're going to get. But if you have a family risk of heart disease or lifestyle factors that put you at risk, increase your odds at better health by supplementing with antioxidants from Maximum Living.

Maximum Living's antioxidant supplement line includes coenzyme Q10, which contains vitamin E (in the form of 400 IU softgel caps), selenium for maximum heart benefit, and a multiple free radical scavenging antioxidant formula that includes not only antioxidant vitamins but also circulation-boosting antioxidant herbals and muscle-strengthening antioxidant amino acids.

Maximum Living's Solu-C (vitamin C) formulas include bioflavonoids for a one-two punch against oxidation. It comes as a tasty chewable for fast and efficient absorption, or an easy-to-swallow capsule that contains green tea for immune boosting and rutin, a bioflavonoid found naturally in food that is credited with strengthening the tiny capillaries of the body. Rutin also helps the body assimilate vitamin C. Add the Solu-C powder to fresh fruit or juice for super health. When you make a fresh cut fruit salad, mix in Solu-C powder for all day freshness and nutrition.

Maximum Living also offers an excellent garlic extract formula that concentrates all the heart-beneficial agents of garlic into a form that's easy to take. It's odorless, too, so you don't have to worry that you'll lose your friends.

RECOVERING FROM THE PARALYZING EFFECTS OF STROKE

David A. Steenblock, M.S., D.O., practicing out of Mission Viejo, California, was the first physician to establish a comprehensive stroke and brain injury rehabilitation facility using Hyperbaric Oxygen Therapy (HBOT) to repair brains damaged from stroke and trauma. The therapy entails putting the patient in a self-enclosed chamber, then pumping in pressurized, rich oxygen, forcing the oxygen into the body's cells.

Strokes are caused by a lack of oxygen to a part of the brain. The symptoms of stroke—drooping mouth, numbness or weakness on one side of the body, difficulty speaking and walking, and uncoordination—are caused by not only a lack of oxygen but also from the swelling of brain tissue and the accumulation of calcium within the damaged nerve cells. HBOT brings oxygen back to starved cells, reduces swelling, and removes the calcium from within the cells—months and even years later.

In one study, 79 patients were treated with HBOT from five months to 10 years after they had their strokes.

Sixty-five percent reported improvement in their quality of life, despite the long delay before treatment.

I have personally seen amazing results with my own eyes. While working with Dr. Steenblock, I saw a young horse trainer who had been kicked in the head by a horse. He couldn't walk, his head lolled against his neck, and he drooled incessantly. His doctors said he would be a vegetable the rest of his life. After HBOT therapy he was able to hold his head up, walk, and feed himself.

I knew an artist in Italy who couldn't hold her paintbrush in paralyzed hands after a stroke. I found her a doctor in Milan who could offer her hyperbaric oxygen therapy. I'll never forget the incredible smile on this tall, beautiful woman when she regained the use of her hands and could continue her artwork. The smile of one person who has recovered makes it all worthwhile—makes my life worthwhile.

THE MEDICAL INDUSTRY EMBRACES HBOT

Researchers at the Memorial Heart Institute at Long Beach Memorial Medical Center in Long Beach, California, conducted laboratory studies on various heart problems and found all were benefited by HBOT. Among its many benefits, the therapy was found to preserve more of the heart's blood-pumping capacity, minimize cell damage and death by reducing fluid accumulation in the injured cells, and even help reduce chest pain.

Currently, hyperbaric chambers are not standard equipment at hospitals and medical centers. The reason is that HBOT adds about $200 to the daily cost of treating a heart attack patient.

Call your local trauma or medical center to learn if they offer hyperbaric oxygen therapy. Or contact the American College for Advancement in Medicine (ACAM) at 800-532-3688; www.acam.org; 23121 Verdugo Drive, Suite 204, Laguna Hills, CA 92653.

THE SAGA CONTINUES

Cholesterol will continue to be a factor in heart disease. Too much clogs the arteries, and not enough starves the brain cells. In the next chapter you will learn what causes cholesterol and how to keep it from being a factor for heart disease.

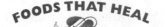

CHAPTER SIX
THE GOOD FATS

> *I believe the essential fatty acids are the primary nutrient missing from the American diet.*
>
> —*Robert C. Atkins, M.D.*

OVER THE PAST FIVE YEARS, Americans have been painfully reminded that the aim of Islamic extremists is to destroy the foundations of free societies and Westerners. There is no compromise possible with assassins whose fanaticism drives them to target our families, friends, and neighbors for death. My brother, who is a Harvard graduate, USMC Lieutenant Colonel Thomas Gillepsie, is proudly serving in Iraq and fully engaged in the battle to defeat terrorism, and defeat it we must.

It's not unlike the battle that's going on inside you! A terrorist, a "sleeper," takes on an unassuming disguise, but is poised to wreak havoc on your insides. His name is LDL Cholesterol. He thickens the blood with cholesterol and clogs the arteries, raising your blood pressure and increasing your risk of a heart attack and arteriosclerosis.

Fortunately, your body has HDL Cholesterol (remember the difference by thinking "Happy" for HDL) as the homeland security force to clear the arteries and protect you from the damage that might occur if LDL is not defeated. Certain foods, nutrients, and supplements will help defeat the sleeper LDL powerful, while other foods increase the HDL security forces.

Follow along as I explain how you can protect yourself.

UNDERSTANDING CHOLESTEROL

Look through any supermarket, and you'll find references to cholesterol on all the labels. Everyone seems obsessed with lowering cholesterol. Cholesterol-lowering drugs have serious side effects, so alternatives should be widely sought. Cholesterol-lowering supplements are among the fastest-growing—sales increased 37 percent in the past year in the natural foods market and 20 percent in the mainstream market.

Before you panic because your doctor said you have high blood cholesterol, take the time to understand what this means. Convention sets the "safe" level of cholesterol for the average adult at 200 mg/dl (milligrams per deciliter). This combines both HDL (high-density lipoproteins) and LDL (low-density lipoproteins) levels. A reading above 200 indicates a potential for developing heart disease, a level of 200 to 239 is borderline, and those over 240 are considered at high risk.

THE BODY NEEDS CHOLESTEROL

Be careful if you choose pharmaceuticals to lower cholesterol levels. Artificially lowering cholesterol is hazardous because we need cholesterol to manufacture sex hormones, vitamin D, DHEA, cell membranes and to protect the body against stress. Lowering cholesterol artificially affects mental acuity and severely disables the ability to cope with physical and mental stress.

The key to lowering cholesterol is to do it naturally, with foods and the nutrients that are found in food. With natural sources, good HDL cholesterol rises while bad LDL is lowered. For instance, supplemental antioxidants—vitamin A, beta carotene, and vitamin C—block cholesterol buildup in the arteries. One study found that vitamin E was 45 percent effective, beta carotene was 90 percent effective, and vitamin C was 95 percent effective in inhibiting the buildup of cholesterol.

Few antioxidant supplements can boast as many potential benefits as grape seed extract. The components in grape seed extract are 20 to 50 times as powerful as vitamins C and E. Grape seed extract contains proanthocyanidins—bioflavonoids that help strengthen and protect cell membranes from free radical damage. The extract also helps prevent oxidation of LDL cholesterol, thus lowering the risk for atherosclerosis and coronary heart disease.

Taking several types of antioxidants are more effective because we need both water-soluble (vitamin C) and fat-soluble (vitamin E) antioxidants. Grape seed extract improves the interaction between them, making them more effective. Maximum Living's Antioxidant formula contains grape seed extract, antioxidant vitamins A, C and E, and other powerful antioxidants that can help prevent cholesterol-related heart problems. It also includes mineral, herbal, and amino acid antioxidants.

CHOLESTEROL-LOWERING COPPER

One of the most satisfying benefits to doing my television program, *Making Healthy Choices*, is the wonderfully interesting research I examine in order to bring new information to each show. Almost every show gives me the opportunity to learn some cutting-edge piece of research that only a privileged few know about. To increase this privileged group, I am only too happy to pass this information on to you.

Richard Kunin, M.D., an orthomolecular psychiatrist and nutrition physician practicing in San Francisco, has been a medical researcher for over 30 years. Dr. Kunin has authored many books, revealing the information gleaned from both experience in his practice and findings from his research. He found the mineral copper to be an answer to the question of high cholesterol. He says that supplementing with copper can lower cholesterol an incredible 800 times more than saturated fat has shown to raise it. And, he says, three out of four Americans are deficient in copper, which means you probably are too. Symptoms of a copper deficiency include heart palpitations, fatigue, depression, *and* high cholesterol.

Zinc and copper need to be taken together because one does not work without the other. For the full benefit and the proper ratios, supplement your minerals in solution with Maximum Living's MineralRich.

FIBER REASONS FOR LOW CHOLESTEROL

Eating more fiber will reduce cholesterol levels. Certain kinds of fiber particularly have been shown to help. Researchers at the Lipid Research Center in Bethesda, Maryland, discovered that the addition of psyllium lowered LDL cholesterol by an incredible 39 percent. They concluded that psyllium, when added to a low-fat diet, works so well it can eliminate the need for cholesterol-lowering drugs.

The research on psyllium is so compelling the FDA has allowed food manufacturers to make this health claim: "Eating soluble fiber from foods such as psyllium as part of a diet low in saturated fat and cholesterol may reduce the risk of heart disease."

We, who have formulated Maximum Living's Hyssop Cleanse, knew this when we formulated our product. It includes not only psyllium and oat bran but also hyssop, which was used in biblical times to cleanse the colon. "Purge me with hyssop, and I shall be clean" (Psalms 51:7).

Maximum Living's Vita Sprout takes fiber from organic vegetables and seed sprouts after harvesting and puts them into capsules or tablets. The kind of vegetables found in this product—carrots, celery, broccoli, and garlic—are excellent sources of cholesterol-lowering fiber.

CHOLESTEROL-FRIENDLY FOOD

The American Heart Association estimates that Americans are getting about half as much fiber in their diet as they need, which is about 30 grams a day.

It isn't coincidence that vegetarians typically have lower blood cholesterol than their meat-eating counterparts. If you don't depend on meat for your entrees, you'll be amazed at the variety of health-giving food from which you can choose. From A to Z, cholesterol-lowering foods are: apples, almonds, avocados, bananas, barley, beans, chili peppers, eggplant, garlic, fruit pectin, oat bran, olive oil, onions, kelp, lentils, peas, green plantains, soybeans, spinach, sweet potatoes, walnuts, yams, and yogurt with active cultures.

Beans, peas, and lentils contain fiber that helps the colon and lowers blood cholesterol. A cup of pinto or navy beans eaten every day was found to lower cholesterol by 19 percent in the subjects of one study. They also favorably affected the ratio of HDL to LDL cholesterol.

The fiber in beans is fermented in the colon into short-chain fatty acids, which are reabsorbed by the body. These acids may help keep the body from making cholesterol. Carbohydrates in the beans are fermented by anaerobic bacteria in the intestines to form hydrogen, carbon dioxide, and methane gases, some of which have to be passed from the system. To remove the troublesome carbohydrates, soak dry beans in water for three to five hours and discard the water before cooking. To retain all the nutrients, use the water but be prepared for the side effects.

Yams or sweet potatoes contain much water-soluble fiber as well as beta carotene, a potent antioxidant that prevents the fats in your body from eating away your insides. Consumed four or five times weekly, yams will contribute to a program of cholesterol control. Japanese researchers rated the fiber in sweet potatoes as best of 28 fruit and vegetable fibers for binding with cholesterol and removing it.

Soybeans and the products derived from them, such as Maximum Living's Nutrition Bites, soy milk, lecithin, and tofu, help break down fatty deposits so they can be flushed from the body more readily. This process also lowers cholesterol. Soybean products seem to work best on patients with high cholesterol— 300 or more. Slightly more than an ounce daily of soybeans has been shown to reduce blood levels of cholesterol by 18 percent. Researchers at the University of Milan, Italy, saw cholesterol levels in their subjects plummet by 15 to 20 percent, simply by having them eat soybeans used in various recipes in place of meat and milk products. Many meat meals can be reproduced by substituting soybean products.

Yogurt is a real winner in lowering cholesterol. Three cups a day have caused cholesterol levels to decline by as much as five to ten percent a week, with the proportion of good guy HDL rising in proportion to LDL. Beware of yogurt substitutes, however. Read the label. Look for yogurt with active cultures. Plain yogurt is your best bet. Use your blender to make a smoothie with it using fresh fruit.

In one study, three medium-sized raw carrots eaten daily was shown to reduce cholesterol by almost eleven percent. That must be how Bugs Bunny does it. He *never* ages!

Chili peppers reduce blood serum cholesterol by suppressing the liver's ability to produce cholesterol. When researchers in Bangkok, Thailand, added freshly ground jalapeno pepper to rice flour noodles, subjects who ate the noodles daily experienced lowered cholesterol and an increased ability to dissolve blood clots.

GARLIC—SUPPLEMENTAL AND FRESH—LOWERS CHOLESTEROL

Garlic doesn't work hanging on the wall or around your neck. You have to eat it. A ration of five fresh raw cloves minced into other foods daily for 25 days has been shown to lower blood serum cholesterol by nearly 10 percent. One doctor fed this amount of garlic to 200 patients with super high blood serum levels.

In almost every patient, cholesterol levels dropped to desired levels.

Scientists at Loma Linda University in California gave supplemental garlic daily to patients with high cholesterol. Six months later these individuals had achieved an average cholesterol reduction of 44 points.

Maximum Living offers the best garlic extract product that needs to be part of any cholesterol-lowering program.

BE FAT SMART

An important issue in cholesterol is fat. Too much of the wrong kind of fat can increase cholesterol levels, but did you realize there is good fat that will lower cholesterol?

Before I continue, let me give you a quick fat lesson. The bad fats are saturated, derived from animals. The good fats go by a variety of names and can be confusing. You hear a great deal about PUFAs, or polyunsaturated fatty acids. PUFAs are a generic term for all the essential fatty acids (EFAs).

We say "essential" because they cannot be made by the body and must be eaten in the diet. They are required for growth, development, and maintenance of cell membranes, including those of the central nervous system. A deficiency of EFAs has been linked to heart disease.

Some of the foods found to lower cholesterol are high in essential fatty acids. These are fish, unroasted nuts and seeds, and the oils from them. The best supplemental sources of essential fatty acids are cod liver oil and borage oil. Borage oil contains linolenic acid, deemed deficient in most of us.

An Australian study found that while both fish and fish oil extracts lower cholesterol, eating fish is more effective. The study, done by the Department of Medicine, University of Western Australia in Perth, found people who ate fish every day for 12 weeks showed a 20 percent reduction in total cholesterol, while those who took fish oil supplements showed a 14 percent reduction. The theory is that something is removed during the purification process of the fish oil that reduces cholesterol.

People living in the Mediterranean have been studied at length due to their low rates of heart disease and cholesterol. In an Israeli study of men in their early twenties, it was found that enrichment of their diet with almonds, avocados, and olive oil reduced their LDL cholesterol by 12 percent. Each of these foods are high in essential fatty acids (EFAs).

I've discussed EFAs in relation to inflammation. They are also important to cholesterol. They provide the kind of cholesterol you need for a healthy mind and a healthy heart. For supplemental omega-3 fatty acid, take Maximum Living's flaxseed oil gel capsules. Flaxseed oil contains 50 to 60 percent omega-3 fatty acids—almost twice as much as fish oil.

Olive oil, almonds, and avocados contain the other kind of EFA: omega-6, found in seeds and seed oils. The best source is gamma-linolenic acid (GLA) from Maximum Living's Borage Oil.

WHAT NOT TO EAT

Now that you know what you should be eating, be prepared to learn what you should NOT be eating. Our nation's epidemic of obesity and heart disease is linked to convenient, processed foods. In the next chapter learn what to avoid and how to keep your need for convenience without sacrificing your health.

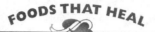
CHAPTER SEVEN

HORMONES, SUGAR, AND OTHER BAD NEWS

> *A beautiful lady*
> *is an accident of nature.*
> *A beautiful old lady*
> *is a work of art.*
>
> —Louis Nizer

I AM A FIRM BELIEVER that as women age, they become more beautiful. It shows in our style and grace—and in our wisdom.

One piece of wisdom all women should have is the knowledge that they are as vulnerable to a heart attack as men. Women account for nearly half of all heart attack deaths, and heart disease is the number-one killer of both women and men.

The fact that women are vulnerable to heart disease is important information that has largely been withheld. For too long, establishment medicine has ignored this risk to women, giving us inadequate information and options. Now, after decades of trusting hormone replacement therapy, women are learning that they've been lied to.

HORMONES AND THE HEARTS OF WOMEN

On July 9, 2002, federal representatives of the National Institutes of Health announced that they had halted a major study on hormone replacement therapy (HRT), because they discovered the long-term use of estrogen and progestin significantly increases the chances of invasive breast cancer, blood clots, and heart attacks. They realized that not only was hormone therapy unlikely to benefit the heart, but after only a year on estrogen and progestin, researchers discovered the risk of heart attack increased by 29 percent, breast cancer by 26 percent, and stroke by 41 percent.

Now that you know HRT can increase your risk of heart problems, you need to know that the symptoms of a heart attack in women can be different than men. For men and women, the most common heart attack symptom is chest pain or discomfort. But other symptoms of a heart attack in women may be ignored, such as shortness of breath, nausea/vomiting, breaking out in a cold sweat, light-headedness, and stomach, arms, back, or jaw pain.

HORMONES IN THE HEARTS OF CATTLE

The same hormones that endanger women using hormone replacement therapy for menopause are fed to animals slaughtered for the dinner table. Those hormones are still detectable in the muscle of animals after they are cooked and can build up in the bodies of humans as they eat them.

Growth hormones given to cattle include estradiol 17, a known carcinogen, as well as synthetic testosterone and progesterone, and the chemicals trenbolone, zeranol, and melengestrol acetate. They are given to cattle and other livestock to promote growth and cause their meat to be tastier for human consumption. The same consequence that makes cattle fat also increases weight and heart problems in the humans eating them.

Members of the European scientific community were so convinced of the dangers of hormonal beef that in 1989 they banned the import of U.S. beef. Hormone residues in meat and meat products can disrupt the natural endocrine equilibrium (hormone balance) that exists within everyone's body. It is now known that any amount of hormones beyond the normal level present in a healthy person is capable of inviting serious health problems, including high blood pressure, heart attack, and stroke.

Treating animals with various types of hormones remains a widely accepted practice within the U.S. meat industry. Hormone pellets are regularly inbred in virtually all cattle.

DON'T GET MILK

Since the early 1970s, study after study has implicated cows' milk and other dairy products as a cause of heart disease and clogged arteries. In a study published in the *International Journal of Cardiology*, researchers studied seven countries with a high consumption of dairy products and found that heart disease mortality rose as milk supply rose. In the *American Journal of Clinical Nutrition*, researchers wrote, "Much evidence suggests that high consumption of full-fat dairy products is likely to increase coronary heart disease risk."

It's not just the fat and cholesterol in dairy products, but also the animal protein and milk carbohydrates that are linked to heart disease. Researchers who studied dietary links to heart disease in 32 countries found that, of all dietary factors studied, milk carbohydrates played the biggest role in the development of heart disease in men over 35, and nonfat milk played the biggest role in the development of coronary heart disease in men over 45. Researchers studying 19 Western countries concluded that heart disease mortality rises as consumption of milk protein rises.

In a study published in the British medical journal *The Lancet*, researchers comparing heart disease death rates with food intake found that the highest correlation was with milk, concluding that milk is the principal dietary culprit in hardened, narrowed arteries and that the problematic portion of milk is its protein.

Dr. Dean Ornish of the University of California at San Francisco has demonstrated that artery blockages can be reversed with a low-fat vegetarian diet instead of expensive and invasive surgeries. The good doctor, himself, switched from nonfat milk to nonfat soy milk, which gives a double benefit. Soy milk has no cholesterol, and soy products can lower cholesterol.

One researcher, Dr. Caldwell Esselstyn from the Cleveland Clinic (the top-rated heart clinic in the U.S.), makes people "heart attack-proof" by putting them on a vegetarian diet.

SUGAR AND SPICE IS NOT SO NICE

Researchers estimate that sugar intake accounts for over 150,000 premature deaths from heart disease yearly in the United States. Indicative of its addictive nature, despite the fact that doctors, nutritionists, and researchers proclaim refined sugar a major nemesis of health, the typical American consumes between 120 and 150 pounds of refined sugar a year. That translates to over one-third of a pound a day—600-plus calories—of teeth-rotting, health-destroying sweetness.

Women's hearts are most affected by sugar. A study by the NASA Langley Research Center, reported in the *Journal of Orthomolecular Medicine*, suggests that sugar is the most important dietary factor related to heart disease in women, while heart disease mortality in men is more heavily related to the consumption of animal fat. Simple sugars raise triglycerides and lower the density of lipoproteins, which are risk factors for cardiovascular disease.

Populations with diets low in refined foods—sugars and simple starches—have a low incidence of heart attacks. Populations with diets high in refined foods have heart attacks and strokes at a higher frequency. When white flour and sugar became cheap and widely available in this century, heart attacks began to occur more frequently.

Over two-thirds of the refined sugar used in this country is added to manufactured food products. In other words, it's hidden in many of the things we buy at the supermarket. Did you know that a tablespoon of ketchup contains a full teaspoon of sugar?

Processed foods such as bread, soup, cereal, cured meat, hot dogs, lunch meat, salad dressing, spaghetti sauce, crackers, mayonnaise, peanut butter, pickles, frozen pizza, canned fruits and vegetables, tomato juice, and a host of other products all contain sugar. This doesn't even take into account the obvious sugary products such as candies, cakes, ice cream, cookies, doughnuts, and soda pop.

SAY NO TO MARGARINE

If you are still eating margarine, where have you been? It is one of the worst things for your heart. You already know saturated fat is bad for you. Saturated fat, such as butter, may increase bad cholesterol, but at least it doesn't touch the good cholesterol. Food processors hydrogenate oils to make them thicker, creamier, and more appetizing to the consumer— hence, margarine. Unfortunately, this process also saturates the oils' fatty acids, changing them to trans fatty acids—hence, poison.

A study conducted in the Netherlands and published in the *New England Journal of Medicine* compared groups of people with diets high in trans fatty acids, or trans fats, with essential fatty acids—such as oil from borage and flaxseed—and saturated fat. The researchers found that the diet high in essential fatty acids had a beneficial effect on blood cholesterol. The diet high in saturated fat raised the level of bad guy LDL cholesterol. But only the diet high in trans fatty acids both increased bad cholesterol and decreased good-guy HDL cholesterol.

A small amount of trans fats comes from dairy products and beef, but the major dietary source is margarine, particularly the hard margarines and shortenings made by hydrogenated plant oils. The Harvard School of Public Health now proclaims that partially hydrogenated vegetable oil, found in margarine and shortening, may be attributed to approximately 30,000 deaths each year.

HEART SMART FOODS

I've been telling you all along some of the foods you should be eating for a healthy heart and cardiovascular system. Keep reading to discover the foods and exercises that are particularly beneficial, and which can literally overcome poor health.

CHAPTER EIGHT

DIET AND EXERCISE— NOT JUST A CLICHÉ

Exercise is a small price to pay for a healthy body and a healthy attitude.

—*Mac Anderson*

AFTER AN EXHAUSTIVE multi-million-dollar health study, the government concluded that people would live longer if they didn't die sooner.

Just like anything else worth the effort, exercise and watching what you eat will pay off with a longer, healthier life.

The principle of a good diet and exercise to prevent or overcome heart disease is not just a cliché, it is valid science. While supplemental nutrition is the most beneficial, you still have to eat. You might as well choose foods that are also nutritionally helpful. Follow along while I give you specifics on exactly what kind of foods and exercise are the most beneficial.

THE MEDITERRANEAN DIET

All the experts state that Mediterranean foods are good for the heart. In 2004 the *Journal of the American Medical Association* proclaimed that a Mediterranean diet can substantially reduce the risk of heart disease and type 2 diabetes and add years of life. Another journal exulted that elderly people who followed this regimen had a death rate more than 50 percent lower than those who did not. It sounds good on the surface but begs the question—which regimen?

There are as many Mediterranean diets as there are Mediterraneans. I've been to Italy—that's in the Mediterranean. But while I was there, I watched them eat white pasta, and I got hooked on tiramisu—a divinely delicious dessert that I'm sure isn't heart healthy.

The geography isn't what's important here, it's the food. While you may have heard of it as such, the Mediterranean diet is not a formal weight-loss diet. It is a principle of culinary eating that inherently benefits the cardiovascular system. It is mainly vegetarian—rich in olive oil, fruits, garlic, vegetables, and whole grains, and low in meat, dairy products, and sweet desserts. The foods typically eaten are low in cholesterol and high in vitamins, flavonoids, minerals, and polyunsaturated fats.

Not coincidentally, the foods of the Mediterranean are ancient, and often referenced in the Bible. They are the foods closest to the earth. I've been saying this since I wrote my book *The Diet Bible* in 1986. Look at a food and ask yourself: did God make this? If so, am I eating it to as close to the way God made it as I possibly can? God's food is as close to nature as possible, retaining the God-given nutrients that feed our God-given bodies.

FOODS OF THE MEDITERRANEAN

For many, the Mediterranean is as comprehensible as the subterranean. Let me help with a short geography lesson. The area is divided into three culinary regions: North African (especially Morocco), eastern Mediterranean (Egypt, Greece, Israel, Lebanon, Syria, and Turkey), and southern European (Italy, France, and Spain). Wine and herbs are central to Southern European cuisine, while spices intricately and boldly flavor North African foods.

Onions, garlic, and tomatoes, surrounded by olive oil, begin many dishes. Eggplants abound, as do squashes, peppers, mushrooms, cucumbers, artichokes, okra, and various greens and lettuces. Legumes too are plentiful: lentils, chickpeas, fava beans in Egypt, green beans in France, and white kidney beans in Tuscany. Fresh herbs include rosemary, basil, cilantro, parsley, mint, dill, fennel, and oregano.

Though the Mediterranean is increasingly fished out and polluted, seafood remains at the core of this cooking heritage. All manner of shellfish erupt magnificently from soups, stews, and pastas. Anchovies, fresh and cured, are widely eaten, as are various white-fleshed fish such sole, flounder, and grouper. Other fish served in the region include swordfish, monkfish, eel, cuttlefish, squid, and octopus. Smaller animals, such as lamb, goats, sheep, pork, rabbit, and fowl, provide most of the meat. Sheep and goats give forth dairy for enzyme-rich yogurts and cheeses. Beef is rare in Mediterranean cuisine, for the land cannot support large herds.

BRINGING THE MEDITERRANEAN HOME

In an ideal world, we enjoy cooking and have as much time as we need to grow our own food and shop for fresh produce. But the reality of life is we seldom have the time or energy to make elaborate, albeit healthy, meals. The next best thing to converting your kitchen into a Greek Taverna is adding foods of the Mediterranean to your diet.

Garlic (Allium sativum)

Garlic is credited in many studies to lower bad cholesterol, raise good cholesterol, and prevent blood platelets from being sticky so they are less able to clump together to form a clot when a blood vessel is injured. It also works to dissolve clots when they do occur.

Garlic was an Egyptian favorite to cure headaches, tumors, and heart problems about 2500 years ago. The plant is so ancient its ancestor is unknown. Garlic was eaten baked whole by the ancient Greeks and fed to the Roman legionaries, who claimed it gave them strength in battle. Garlic may have saved people from the plague during the Middle Ages, and garlic-eating priests who tended the sick fared better than those less fond of the herb.

For your eating pleasure, look for garlic heads that are firm with plenty of dry, papery covering. Heads that are showing signs of sprouting are past their prime. As with all ingredients for cooking, buy the best garlic you can afford. I recommend organic garlic if at all possible.

In general with garlic, the finer the chop the stronger the taste. Crushed garlic has the strongest taste of all. When cooked, whole garlic has a much milder and rather sweet taste. Garlic added at the end of cooking will give a stronger taste than garlic prepared the same way but added earlier.

To get the cardiovascular benefits of garlic, eat one

or two cloves daily. A ration of five fresh raw cloves minced into other foods daily for 25 days has been shown to lower blood serum cholesterol by nearly 10 percent. Try garlic paste squeezed from roasted garlic. You can put it into a small mustard jar and use it like mayonnaise. There is no odor as long as it is roasted whole. Garlic's odor comes from it being chopped raw. Whole garlic is also available pickled, in jars. Chewing raw parsley can help with unpleasant garlic breath.

Olive Oil

It's official. Under a "qualified health claim" granted by the Food and Drug Administration (FDA), bottles of olive oil can now boast what proponents of the Mediterranean style of eating have long contended—olive oil helps reduce the risk of heart disease. That's because olive oil contains monounsaturated fatty acids, which lower bad LDL cholesterol. Olive oil also appears to reduce the inflammation tied to artery damage, and it seems to keep the inner lining of arteries calm and less likely to contract in a dangerous way.

Eat olive oil raw in salads, with whole grain bread or baked in foods. Never fry anything. It not only kills nutrients, but the resultant chemical reaction can produce carcinogens.

Most domestic olive oil comes from California, with imported oils from France, Greece, Italy, and Spain. All olive oils are graded in accordance with the degree of acidity they contain. The best are cold-pressed, a chemical-free process that involves only pressure, which produces a natural level of low acidity. Extra virgin olive oil is made from the first cold-pressing and is only one percent acid. It's considered the finest and fruitiest of the olive oils and is therefore also the most expensive. In general, the deeper the color, the more intense the olive flavor.

Products labeled simply olive oil (once called pure olive oil) contain a combination of refined olive oil and virgin or extra virgin oil. The new light olive oil contains the same amount of beneficial monounsaturated fat as regular olive oil...and it also has exactly the same number of calories.

Olive oil can be stored in a cool dark place for up to six months. It can be refrigerated, in which case it will last up to a year. Chilled olive oil becomes cloudy and too thick to pour. However, it will clear and become liquid again when brought to room temperature.

Tomatoes

Call it the revenge of the tomatoes. Until the 1800s Americans considered tomatoes a poisonous fruit, either rarely eaten or boiled for hours to destroy its "toxins." Recently scientists have discovered spectacular secrets in tomatoes—various disease-fighting antioxidants, including the red pigment lycopene and an anti-clotting agent known as "P3 tomato factor." These discoveries have transformed the tomato into a hot health food, increasingly believed to help prevent and even reverse disease.

Researchers in Australia discovered that tomato juice acts as an effective blood thinner, working to break up blood clots or prevent the clumping of blood cells. Study benefactors drank eight ounces of tomato juice every day for three weeks. If you choose canned tomato juice, pick the variety with no MSG, usually labeled as "natural flavoring."

Tomatoes can make you less prone to clogged arteries and heart disease. Dramatic new evidence from Finland shows that middle-aged men with low lycopene are three times more apt to suffer heart attacks or strokes and 18 percent more likely to have narrowed carotid (neck) arteries. One reason may be that tomatoes help detoxify bad LDL cholesterol, hindering plaque building. In one test, eating 60 milligrams of lycopene daily (the amount in 1-1/2 cups tomato sauce or 2.2 pounds of fresh tomatoes) for three months reduced LDL cholesterol by 14 percent.

An aspirin-like substance in the yellow jelly around tomato seeds helps thwart blood clots, according to Scottish research. The amount in only four tomatoes reduced clot-provoking blood stickiness by a surprising 72 percent.

To get the greatest benefit:

- Eat at least five weekly servings of tomato based foods.
- Eat tomatoes cooked and prepared with a little olive oil. Heating helps release lycopene, and you get the most lycopene in concentrated, processed products, such as tomato paste and sauce, canned tomatoes, juice, and soup. Still, Americans get half their lycopene from raw tomatoes. In new tests at Ohio State University, over a two-week period, blood lycopene was raised 192 percent by a daily serving of tomato sauce, 122 percent by tomato soup, and 92 percent by tomato juice. Other research shows that adding olive oil to tomatoes increases lycopene absorption.
- Eat a variety. Lycopene isn't the sole tomato power. For example, tomato soup has more antioxidant

activity than can be attributed to lycopene alone, meaning it contains other antioxidants. Raw tomatoes are lower in lycopene but are still good at combatting blood clots.

Figs—A Biblical High Fiber Fruit

Much of the fruit eaten in the Mediterranean is high in fiber, such as figs, apples, raisins, and plums, but figs have the most fiber. The fiber in figs is both soluble and insoluble. Both types of fiber are important for good health.

Figs have nutrients especially important for today's busy lifestyles. One quarter-cup serving of dried figs provides five grams of fiber. Figs have no fat, no sodium, and no cholesterol. Recent research has shown that figs also have a high quantity of polyphenol antioxidants. Figs have a notable amount of protein and abundant calcium, magnesium, phosphorus, and potassium. They are a good source of the indigestible food fiber lignin.

There was a fig tree in the Garden of Eden, and in fact, the fig is the most talked about fruit in the Bible. Whether a fig was the forbidden fruit is debatable, but it is definite that a fig tree provided the first clothing: ". . . the eyes of both of them were opened, and they knew that they were naked; and they sewed fig leaves together, and made themselves aprons" (Genesis 3:7).

Pliny, the Roman writer (A.D. 52–113), said, "Figs are restorative. They increase the strength of young people, preserve the elderly in better health, and make them look younger with fewer wrinkles."

When buying figs, look for plump soft fresh figs with skin that is green, brown, or purple, depending on the variety. As figs ripen, the pectin in their cell walls dissolves, and the figs grow softer to the touch. Choose dried figs in tightly sealed airtight packages. Avoid fresh figs that smell sour. The odor indicates that the sugars in the fig have fermented and the fruit is spoiled.

Refrigerate fresh figs. Dried figs can be stored in the refrigerator or at room temperature; either way, wrap them tightly in an air- and moisture-proof container. Dried figs may keep for several months.

Whenever you increase your intake of fiber, always drink plenty of purified water—at least eight glasses a day.

Almonds

Almonds were known to the people of Israel very early in Bible history. Almonds were included as a gift from Jacob/Israel to the Prime Minister of Egypt. "And their father Israel said unto them, If it must be so now, do this; take of the best fruits in the land in your vessels, and carry down the man a present, a little balm, and a little honey, spices, and myrrh, nuts, and almonds" (Genesis 43:11).

Almonds are high in bioavailable (easily absorbed by the body) magnesium as well as rich in monounsaturated fat. Almonds also contain vitamin E, helpful in avoiding blood clots. A one-ounce handful of almonds provides 7.3 milligrams of vitamin E.

In a study reported in the *Journal of Nutrition*, almonds were found to reduce triglycerides (the body's main fat-carrying particle), total and LDL cholesterol by up to 14 percent, and increase HDL—good—cholesterol by six percent. Raw or roasted almonds were found to influence cholesterol better than almond butter, although almond butter does help increase good cholesterol.

Dr. David Jenkins, Faculty of Medicine, University of Toronto, Canada, found that patients who ate about one ounce of almonds each day lowered their LDL cholesterol significantly. There was an even greater decrease for those who ate about two handfuls of almonds per day.

C-reactive protein, the marker that indicates inflammation, was found to be reduced in a diet that includes almonds, according to an article in the *Journal of the American Medical Association*.

Try a handful of almonds as a snack or sprinkled on a salad or a pasta or rice dish.

Have you ever tried marzipan? It's candy made of ground almonds. You can buy tubes of it in the supermarket without sugar. It's delicious without any sweetener.

Eat almonds to "buy American." Approximately 6,000 almond growers in California produce more than 75 percent of all the world's almonds. That's good enough for me!

Whole Grains

Whole grains are made up of all parts of the grain—the bran (or fiber-rich outer layer), the endosperm (middle part), and the germ (the nutrient-rich inner part). When grains are milled, or refined, the bran and germ portions are removed. As man's diet got "civilized," whole grain, nutritional bread was replaced by milled flour, devoid of fiber, vitamins, and minerals. It got so bad food processors were required to supplement nutrients back into bread to keep us from becoming sick.

When you eat whole grain foods, you get the nutritional benefits of the entire grain, including heart healthy fiber. In chapter 6, I talked about lowering cholesterol with fiber. High intake of dietary fiber—particularly from grains—is linked to a lower risk of heart disease in a number of large studies that followed people for many years. In a Harvard study of over 40,000 male health professionals, researchers found that a high total dietary fiber intake was associated with a 40 percent lower risk of coronary heart disease. A related Harvard study of female nurses produced quite similar findings.

Fiber intake has also been linked with the metabolic syndrome, a constellation of factors that increases the chances of developing heart disease and diabetes. These factors include high blood pressure, high insulin levels, excess weight (especially around the abdomen), high levels of triglycerides, and low levels of HDL (good) cholesterol. Several studies suggest that higher intake of fiber may somehow ward off this increasingly common syndrome.

Identifying whole grains in your food sources can be tricky. Out of all the breads available in U.S. supermarkets, only whole wheat bread is really whole grain. Cornmeal is rarely whole grain. Quinoa and oatmeal are whole grains. Bulgur and couscous sometimes are and sometimes aren't. The bagel store sells "whole grain" bagels, but are they really whole grain?

Check out food labels to help you choose more whole grain foods each day. Look at both the "Ingredient List" and the "Nutrition Facts" panel and try to choose foods that list a whole grain as the first ingredient. Also look for a "whole grain" claim on other parts of the package labels. For qualifying foods, the government has approved a health claim that states: "Diets rich in whole grain foods, and other plant foods and low in total fat, saturated fat, and cholesterol, may help reduce the risk of heart disease and certain cancers."

Legumes

Legumes are a family of plants that are identified by their seed-bearing pods. They are all the common beans (black, pinto, kidney, and white), lentils, fava beans, chickpeas (garbanzos), and dried split peas.

Legumes are powerhouses of protein, carbohydrates, vitamins, minerals, and phytochemicals (plant chemicals). Legumes are an excellent source of fiber. For example, in 1/4 cup of dried black beans there are 15 grams of fiber and 0 percent fat.

Researchers from Tulane University School of Public Health and Tropical Medicine in New Orleans identified a reduced risk of coronary heart disease with increased legume consumption. The Tulane researchers concluded legumes protected against heart disease because of the protective properties of calcium, fiber, folate, magnesium, potassium, and copper. The Tulane study found that those eating legumes had lower systolic blood pressure, less hypertension, lower levels of total cholesterol and hypercholesterolemia, and less diabetes, in spite of having eaten more fat.

Plan ahead when serving legumes. Add a pinch of cayenne and nutmeg; it's a delicious addition to beans. Allow time for them to cook; they will need little attention while slow cooking. Just add water if they get a little dry. Try putting some in a Crock-Pot in the morning before you go to work. When you come home, not only does your house smell wonderful from the onions and garlic, but dinner is almost ready to be served. All you have to do now is round out the meal with a vegetable, bread, fruit, and beverage, and you have a tasty, nutritious, heart-healthy meal.

Fish

In chapter 6, I discussed the value of fish oil—omega-3 fatty acids—but now it's time to talk about eating fish. Certain fish offer the health value of not only EFAs but also certain nutrients known to benefit the heart, circulation, and the heart muscle. Salmon seems to be the star performer for the heart.

The most potent antioxidant for the heart, coenzyme Q10, is found in codfish, mackerel, salmon, and sardines. For fatty acids, the darker the fish, the better. Bluefish, salmon, and other dark-hued fish contain the most omega-3.

The most beneficial and active of omega-3 fatty acids are eicosapentaenoic acid (EPA) and docosahexaenoic acid (DHA). Fatty fish such as salmon and herring are good sources of EPA and DHA.

Never fry fish. Not only is the oil it is fried in bad for you at high heat, but the oils in fish chemically mutate and become carcinogenic. Instead, bake, broil, grill, or poach fish. Use spices low in salt and additives. Baste with olive oil and flavor with lemon juice.

EXERCISING YOUR WAY TO A HEALTHY HEART

Wesley Miller was a walking medicine cabinet after undergoing triple-bypass surgery in 1994. By late

2001, he was on 16 drugs, including Lipitor for high cholesterol, Glucotrol for diabetes, and three pills to lower his blood pressure. He couldn't walk from his front doorstep to the mailbox without doubling over in chest pain. At one point, tests showed the blockages were back and that his arteries were too damaged to risk another operation. He thought he might die.

But Miller, now 65, discovered a lifesaver—not more drugs but a program of daily exercise, stress reduction, group support, and a diet very low in fat and high in vegetables and whole grains. After seven weeks on this low-tech form of medicine, recommended by his doctor and designed by California's Dr. Dean Ornish, Wes Miller started to get better. The angina attacks faded. In eight months he lost 40 pounds. His blood pressure eased off, his cholesterol level fell from 243 to 110, and his blood sugar normalized.

A gerontologist and heart specialist studying the long-lived Soviet Abkhasians found that although they often suffer mild heart attacks, exercise has so strengthened their heart-lung systems that they don't know it. Their superior oxygen supply to the heart overcomes local blockages that would be crippling or fatal to an average person.

Researchers in Perth, Australia, using a new type of ultrasound that can produce an image of artery walls, found overweight kids as young as six years of age with hardening of the arteries. They set out to see if exercise alone could reverse it. It did—in just eight weeks.

And what kind of exercise did the kids do? They lifted weights. They gained weight, but it was because they converted their fat into muscle. And when they exercised, they stretched their arteries, which helped loosen the plaque. The increased blood flow from the strenuous exercise helped move the plaque away.

If you need to lose weight and gain strength, try weight-bearing exercise. Three one-hour workouts at low intensity burn off fat better than six 30-minute sessions at high intensity.

If you hate heavy, stressful workouts, I have good news. Strenuous exercise is not the best idea. It increases free radical activity, stresses the joints, and as you breathe heavily, you take in more pollutants faster. Science is now saying it is moderate exercise that prevents illness, increases health, and promotes mental vitality.

While losing weight can help heart health, exercise to lose weight isn't necessary to see health benefits. Researchers from Duke University reported in the *New England Journal of Medicine* that moderate exercise produces benefits to the cardiovascular system—even if it is not enough to see weight loss. The equivalent of walking 12 miles per week (2 miles a day for six days) showed significant benefit—the same benefit as jogging 20 miles per week.

Exercise is the unanimously uncontested age reverser. It is credited with reversing heart disease, diabetes, hypertension, osteoporosis, depression, and mental problems. It increases circulation, strength, bone mass, immune system function, and mental vitality.

You may not be 86 yet, but it's comforting to know that even at that late hour, you can still reverse the effects of having been a couch potato. My workout buddy, Edna Markus, lifts weights and rides a stationary bicycle. She can push 50 pounds off her chest and lift 30 pounds with both legs. Edna is 86 years old.

Edna's family was prepared to place her into long-term nursing care. Instead, they enrolled her in a special seniors' weight-training program three times a week. Now she lives independently in her senior apartment complex surrounded by friends who seek her out because she makes them feel good about themselves.

Of course, what constitutes moderate exercise is different for everyone. To me, moderate exercise is a game of tennis, racquetball, or golf. What is important, no matter what your age, is tailoring your exercise to your fitness level and enjoying what you do.

A MERRY HEART DOETH GOOD LIKE A MEDICINE

There is an anatomy of joy, says William Fry, a Stanford University psychiatrist and pioneer in laughter research. The muscles of the abdomen, neck, and shoulders rapidly tighten and relax, the heart speeds up, the blood pressure rises, and breathing becomes spasmodic and deeper. It happens whenever we let ourselves go in dancing, running, and jumping for the fun of it. It also occurs when we laugh so hard our whole body is convulsed. "One hundred laughs is equal to ten minutes of rowing," says Dr. Fry. "Sustained hilarity is among the more agreeable forms of aerobics."

The most astonishing evidence of laughter's power comes from a 1997 study of 48 heart attack patients. Half watched comedic television shows for 30 minutes every day, and the other half watched dramas. After a year, ten patients in the drama control group had suffered repeat heart attacks, compared with only two in the same group that watched comedy shows.

Researchers suggest that we need a minimum of twelve laughs a day to stay healthy. Laugh loud, and laugh often. It will keep your heart healthy.

MAUREEN SALAMAN continues to formulate leading-edge products based on the latest scientific research and highest production standards to ensure the natural force and power of the nutrients are retained. This expertise and her leadership are a vital part of the Maximum Living company.

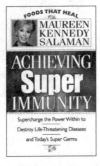

Also in this Series

#610 / $7.95

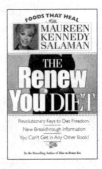

Also in this Series

#620 / $7.95

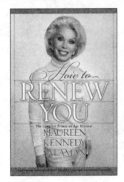
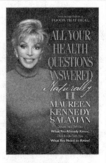
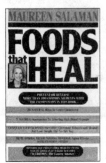

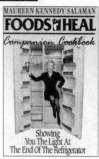
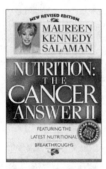
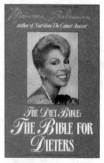